THE PALEO DIET

COOKBOOK

FOR

NEWBIES AND BEGINNERS

BY

Dr. Christen Zimmermann

Table of Contents

INTRODUCTION

A paleo diet is a dietary plan based on foods similar to what might have been eaten during the Paleolithic era, which dates from approximately 2.5 million to 10,000 years ago.

A paleo diet typically includes lean meats, fish, fruits, vegetables, nuts and seeds — foods that in the past could be obtained by hunting and gathering. A paleo diet limits foods that became common when farming emerged about 10,000 years ago. These foods include dairy products, legumes and grains.

Other names for a paleo diet include Paleolithic diet, Stone Age diet, hunter-gatherer diet and caveman diet.

Purpose

The aim of a paleo diet is to return to a way of eating that's more like what early humans ate. The diet's reasoning is that the human body is genetically mismatched to the modern diet that emerged with farming practices — an idea known as the discordance hypothesis.

Farming changed what people ate and established dairy, grains and legumes as additional staples in the human diet. This relatively late and rapid change in diet, according to the hypothesis, outpaced the body's ability to adapt. This mismatch is believed to be a contributing factor to the prevalence of obesity, diabetes and heart disease today.

WHY YOU MIGHT FOLLOW A PALEO DIET

You might choose to follow a paleo diet because you:

- Want to lose weight or maintain a healthy weight
- Want help planning meals

Details of a paleo diet

Recommendations vary among commercial paleo diets, and some diet plans have stricter guidelines than others. In general, paleo diets follow these guidelines.

WHAT TO EAT

- Fruits
- Vegetables
- Nuts and seeds
- Lean meats, especially grass-fed animals or wild game
- Fish, especially those rich in omega-3 fatty acids, such as salmon, mackerel and albacore tuna
- Oils from fruits and nuts, such as olive oil or walnut oil

WHAT TO AVOID

- Grains, such as wheat, oats and barley

- Legumes, such as beans, lentils, peanuts and peas
- Dairy products
- Refined sugar
- Salt
- Potatoes
- Highly processed foods in general

A typical day's menu

Here's a look at what you might eat during a typical day following a paleo diet:

- Breakfast. Broiled salmon and cantaloupe.
- Lunch. Broiled lean pork loin and salad (romaine, carrot, cucumber, tomatoes, walnuts and lemon juice dressing).
- Dinner. Lean beef sirloin tip roast, steamed broccoli, salad (mixed greens, tomatoes, avocado, onions, almonds and lemon juice dressing), and strawberries for dessert.
- Snacks. An orange, carrot sticks or celery sticks.

The diet also emphasizes drinking water and being physically active every day.

Results

A number of randomized clinical trials have compared the paleo diet to other eating plans, such as the Mediterranean Diet or the Diabetes Diet. Overall, these trials suggest that a paleo diet may provide some benefits when compared with diets of fruits, vegetables, lean meats, whole grains, legumes and low-fat dairy products. These benefits may include:

• More weight loss

• Improved glucose tolerance

• Better blood pressure control

• Lower triglycerides

• Better appetite management

However, longer trials with large groups of people randomly assigned to different diets are needed to understand the long-term, overall health benefits and possible risks of a paleo diet.

QUESTIONS ABOUT PALEO DIETS

Concerns or questions about the paleo diet include both food selection and the underlying hypothesis.

Dietary concerns

A paleo diet is rich in vegetables, fruits and nuts — all elements of a healthy diet.

The primary difference between the paleo diet and other healthy diets is the absence of whole grains and legumes, which are considered good sources of fiber, vitamins and other nutrients. Also absent from the diet are dairy products, which are good sources of protein and calcium.

These foods not only are considered healthy but also are generally more affordable and accessible than such foods as wild game, grass-fed animals and nuts. For some people, a paleo diet may be too expensive.

QUESTIONS ABOUT THE PALEO DIET HYPOTHESIS

Researchers have argued that the underlying hypothesis of the paleo diet may oversimplify the story of how humans adapted to changes in diet. Arguments for a more-complex understanding of the evolution of human nutritional needs include the following:

• Variations in diet based on geography, climate and food availability — not only the transition to farming — also would have shaped the evolution of nutritional needs.

• Archaeological research has demonstrated that early human diets may have included wild grains as much as 30,000 years ago — well before the introduction of farming.

• Genetic research has shown that notable evolutionary changes continued after the Paleolithic era, including diet-related changes, such as an increase in the number of genes related to the breakdown of dietary starches.

THE BOTTOM LINE

A paleo diet may help you lose weight or maintain your weight. It may also have other beneficial health effects. However, there are no long-term clinical studies about the benefits and potential risks of the diet.

You might be able to achieve the same health benefits by getting enough exercise and eating a balanced, healthy diet with a lot of fruits and vegetables.

TURMERIC SAUTEED GREENS

Turmeric has been used in cuisines all over the world for centuries as it has all kinds of natural benefits like being an anti-depressant and having natural anti-inflammatory properties. By just adding a little to dishes you enjoy you'll receive tons of healing powers you and your family may need more than you know.

Ingredients

• 1 tablespoon olive oil

• 3 garlic cloves, minced

• 1 2-inch piece fresh turmeric

• 2 bunches kale, spinach, or swiss chard, thinly sliced

• 1/4 teaspoon kosher salt

• 2 tablespoons water

Preparation

1. Heat oil in a large sauce pan over medium heat.

2. Add garlic and turmeric and saute for 30 seconds.

3. Add kale and salt and saute for 1 minute.

4. Add water to the pan and cook stirring until the greens are just wilted and serve.

Spiced Carrot Cauliflower Soup

The flavorful spice combination of curry, cinnamon, and garam marsala partnered with the sweet taste of the carrots and creamy texture of the cooked cauliflower makes for one of the most flavorful soups you could imagine. While you're making it, let your kids smell and taste the spices. You can also let them shake them into the pot and even use a hand blender (pretty kid-safe with adult supervision) to puree everything together. They will really feel a part of the fun and it's a great way to introduce kids to the incredible world of spices.

Ingredients

- 1 tablespoon olive oil
- 1 small onion, chopped
- 5 cups warm water
- 2 tablespoons vegetable bouillon*
- 1 head cauliflower, chopped (about 4 cups)
- 3 cups peeled and chopped carrots (about 8 medium carrots)

• 1 1/2 teaspoons curry powder

• 1 teaspoon ground cinnamon

• 1 teaspoon garam masala

• 1 teaspoon kosher salt

• *I like to use Organic Better Than Bouillon instead of the cubes

Preparation

1. Heat the oil in a large saucepan over medium heat and cook the onions for 3 minutes, or until soft.

2. Dissolve the vegetable bouillon in the water and add to the pot.

3. Add the remaining ingredients to the pot and stir to combine.

4. Bring to a boil, cover, and reduce heat to simmer for 15-20 minutes, or until the vegetables are fork tender.

5. Using an immersion blender or standing blender, puree all of the ingredients until smooth.

Turkey Zucchini Burgers with Yogurt-Sumac Sauce

The zucchini gives these burgers a little extra texture and moistness while plumping them up with a vegetable for those kids who have an aversion to zucchini. If you've got tons of zucchini growing in your garden you need to make these beauties! They're the perfect summertime meal to get you excited for the season no matter where your inspiration comes from!

Ingredients

- For the burgers:
- 1-pound ground turkey, light or dark meat
- 1 large zucchini, coarsely grated
- 3 scallions, thinly sliced
- 1 large egg
- 2 tablespoons chopped mint
- 2 tablespoon chopped cilantro
- 2 garlic cloves, minced
- 1 teaspoon ground cumin

• 1 teaspoon kosher salt

• olive oil, for greasing the pan

• 8 mini hamburger buns

• For the yogurt sauce:

• 1 cup greek yogurt

• 1 teaspoon grated lemon zest

• 1 tablespoon lemon juice

• 1 garlic clove, minced

• 1 tablespoon olive oil

• 2 teaspoons sumac

• 1/2 teaspoon kosher salt

Preparation

1. In a large bowl combine first 9 ingredients. Mix well. With dampened hands form the mixture into burgers about 1 inch thick. You can do small slider size or regular size burgers.

2. In a large saute pan or stove top grill over medium, add 1-2 tablespoons olive oil and add the burger patties. Cook burgers 3-4 minutes on each side for small slider burgers or 5-6 minutes on each side for larger burgers.

3. Place all the sauce ingredients in a small bowl and stir to combine.

4. Place the burgers on buns and top with the yogurt-sumac sauce.

Salmon Sheet Pan Dinner

Not only is this Salmon Sheet Pan Dinner gorgeous to look at it's even better to taste. Make it for a party or a night home with the family hen you want to spend as much time out of the kitchen as possible so you can maximize relaxing and having fun!

Ingredients

• 1 1/2 cups cherry tomatoes

• 1 large fennel bulb, sliced lengthwise into steaks

• 1 zucchini, cut into coins

• olive oil

• 2 lemons, halved

• 1 1/2 pounds salmon filet, whole or cut into filets

• kosher salt, to taste

Preparation

1. Preheat oven to 450 degrees F.

2. Place the first 5 ingredients on a sheet pan and toss with olive oil to coat and salt to taste. Distribute the

vegetables around the pan in a single layer and bake for 10 minutes.

3. Remove the sheet pan from the oven and push some of the vegetables to the side to make space for the salmon fillets. Season the salmon with salt and bake for 12-15 additional minutes (depending on the thickness of your salmon fillets).

4. Turn the broiler on for 2 minutes or until the vegetables are golden.

5. Place salmon and vegetables on a plate and offer a lemon half for s�ueezing over fish and vegetables.

Spiced Chicken with Olives and Lemon

Spiced Chicken with Olives and Lemon is super healthy and a �uick weeknight meal full of flavor that everyone will love.

Ingredients

- 2 tablespoons olive oil
- 1 large onion, halved, thinly sliced
- 2 cloves garlic, minced
- 1 teaspoon salt, divided
- 2 lemons, 1 cut into 8 wedges �uartered and deseeded and one juiced
- 1 tablespoon paprika
- 2 teaspoons ground cumin
- 1 teaspoon ground cinnamon
- 1 teaspoon ground ginger
- 1 15 ounce can low-sodium chicken broth
- 4 chicken breasts, boneless and skinless

• 1 10 ounce jar Castelvetrano Olives, pitted and reserving all the juice

Preparation

1. Heat oil in large skillet over medium heat, add onion and garlic, sprinkle with 1/2 tsp salt and saute until golden, about 4-5 minutes.

2. Add the juice of one lemon and next 5 ingredients; stir 1 minute. Add broth and reserved olive juice and bring to boil.

3. Sprinkle chicken with remaining 1/2 tsp salt add to skillet. Add the remaining 8 lemon wedges and olives. Cover, reduce heat to low, and simmer 25-35 minutes or until chicken is cooked through, turning occasionally. Transfer chicken to platter and serve.

Crock Pot Ribs

Only two basic ingredients- pork ribs and your favorite barbecue sauce added right to your Crock Pot to simmer for hours making a meal that will seem like it took hours to prepare (but didn't). For this Rewind Wednesday you're going to be a culinary hero making a dish that's going to be on your menu plan for months to come!

Ingredients

• 1 3-4 pound country style pork ribs, also known as baby back ribs (about 2 racks)

• 1 Tsp kosher salt

• 1 Cup BBQ Sauce plus additional for serving (my favorite is Smokin Willie's)

Preparation

1. Place ribs in a crock pot and sprinkle both sides with salt.

2. Pour BBQ sauce over the ribs and coat the ribs WELL with the sauce.

3. Cover the slow cooker (aka crock pot) and cook on low heat for 8-10 hours.

4. Baste with BBQ sauce if desired and serve.

Stir-Fried Chicken in Lettuce Cups

Salad may be a tough sell for some little ones, but these lettuce cups are kid friendly and a whole new way for them of looking at leafy greens. They're crunchy, and in combination with the stir-fried chicken with herbs and a slightly sweet sauce it's really something special.

Ingredients

- 1/4 cup low sodium soy sauce
- 2 tablespoons honey
- 2 tablespoons cilantro, chopped
- 1 tablespoons oil
- 1 small onion, diced
- 1 bell pepper, any color, chopped
- 1 garlic clove, minced
- 1 teaspoon ginger, minced
- 1 pound ground chicken or turkey
- 1/4 teaspoon kosher salt
- 8 bibb or iceberg lettuce cups

Preparation

1. Combine soy sauce, honey, and cilantro in a bowl and set aside.

2. Using a large saute pan, cook the onion in 1 tbsp of oil over medium heat for 2 minutes.

3. Add the bell pepper and cook an additional 2 minutes.

4. Add the garlic and ginger and cook for 1 minute then add the chicken or turkey to the pan and saute for an additional 7 minutes or until cooked through.

5. Stir in the soy sauce mixture, salt and cook for 2 minute or until juices evaporate.

6. Serve in lettuce cups (to eat then just roll the lettuce around the stir fried chicken and eat them like a burrito).

Southern Style Pork Tenderloin

Southern Style Pork Tenderloin is smoky, sweet, and tangy all in one. This is the perfect summer grilling recipe.

Ingredients

• 1/4 cup bourbon

• 1/4 cup soy sauce

• 1/4 cup brown sugar

• 1/4 cup dijon mustard

• 3 tbsp olive oil

• 1 tablespoon finely chopped fresh ginger

• 3 garlic cloves, minced

• 2 whole pork tenderloins, approximately 2 pounds total, trimmed

Preparation

1. Place the first seven ingredients in a bowl and whisk to combine. Pour into a large zipper bag or glass container large enough to hold the pork tenderloins and marinate overnight or up to 2 days.

2. Preheat a grill to high heat, and oil the grates.

3. Remove tenderloins from the bag, reserving the marinade, and grill for 14-15 minutes, turning halfway through or until the internal temperature is 140°F. Remove from heat and set meat aside to rest for 5-10 minutes to allow the juices to rest and redistribute.

4. While the meat is resting, place the marinade in a small pan. Bring to a boil, reduce to a simmer and cook for 10 minutes.

5. Slice the tenderloin on a bias and serve with the sauce if desired.

Roast Chicken with Caramelized Lemons, Cherry Tomatoes and Olives

This Roast Chicken with Caramelized Lemons, Cherry Tomatoes and Olives has �uickly become one of my trusted, tried and true dinner entrees for a plethora of reasons. It's super simple (hello only 5 ingredients and only one pan) and incredibly delicious. This is one of the best Roast Chicken recipes you'll try this week!

Ingredients

- 1 tablespoon vegetable or canola oil
- 4 chicken breasts, bone in and skin on
- 1 teaspoon kosher salt
- 1 lemon cut in half
- 1/2 cup pitted black olives
- 1/2 cup cherry tomatoes
- handful of thyme (about 8-10 stems)

Preparation

1. Preheat oven to 450°F.

2. Heat the oil in an oven-proof skillet over medium-high heat.

3. Pat the chicken breasts dry, make sure they are very dry, and sprinkle the top with the salt.

4. Place the chicken breasts, skin side down, in the heated oil and sear for 5 minutes, or until skin is crisp and golden brown.

5. Flip the chicken over. Add the lemon, olives, tomatoes and thyme to the skillet and transfer to the oven.

6. Roast for 25 minutes, or until chicken is cooked through.

Simple Sauteed Collard Greens

Ingredients

• 1 slice thick-cut bacon, diced

• 1 bunch collard greens

• 2 garlic cloves, minced

• 1/2 teaspoon kosher salt

Preparation

1. Place the bacon in a sauté pan over medium-low heat and cook for 5 minutes to render as much fat as possible.

2. While the bacon is cooking, remove the stems from the collard greens, and thinly slice the leaves across.

3. Add the garlic to the pan and cook for 1 minute. Add the greens and salt, stir well to coat the greens with the bacon fat, reduce heat to low, and cook for 5 minutes, until wilted, stirring occasionally. If you like them softer, cook for 10 minutes.

Slow Cooker Bone Broth

I've always been fascinated by food trends. The past few years it's been all about kale and why it's the only vegetable you should be eating in salads, smoothies, baked as chips and more. But just the other day I read a lengthy article about an author who was breaking up with kale. Should you really break up with healthy foods?!

Ingredients

- 10-12 pounds beef bones
- 2 tablespoons apple cider vinegar
- 2 onions, peeled and �uartered
- 2 carrots, peeled and cut in half
- 2 celery stalks, cut in half
- 2 bay leaves
- 2 tablespoons peppercorns
- 4 stems parsley
- 1 teaspoon kosher salt

Preparation

1. Place the beef bones in the slow cooker, and place the remaining ingredients on top.

2. Add enough water to the slow cooker to cover everything.

3. Cover, set the slow cooker to high, and cook for 24-72 hours.

4. Strain the li�uid, place in the refrigerator to cool, remove the solidified fat from the top, and use as desired.

Seafood Stew

Even as a kid I loved seafood. We're talking clams, mussels, squid, you name it, I love it. I know at least one of my kids came out of the womb with the seafood gene. On any given day since she was a baby, Chloe would either be yelling "more calamari" across a restaurant or asking the seafood vendors at our farmers market, Marilyn and Eileen, for baby clams, whole octopus or smoked salmon. These are the moments I realize the apple doesn't fall far from the tree.

Ingredients

- 1 tablespoon oil
- 1 large onion, diced
- 6 garlic cloves, minced
- 1 cup dry white wine
- 1 28-ounce can diced tomatoes
- 1 cup clam juice
- 1 bay leaf
- 1 teaspoon kosher salt

• 1/2 pound mussels

• 1/2 pound clams

• 1/2 pound shrimp, peeled and deveined

• 1/2 pound calamari, sliced into rings

• 1/4 cup minced parsley, for garnish, optional

Preparation

In a large stock pot, heat oil over medium high heat.

Add the onions and cook for 3-4 minutes, until tender. Add garlic and sauté for another minute.

Add the wine, tomatoes, clam juice, bay leaf and salt. Bring to a boil, then reduce heat to medium and simmer for 20 minutes.

Add in all the seafood at once and stir to combine. Cook until shrimp is pink and cooked through and mussels and clams have opened, about 5-7 minutes.

Garnish with parsley if desired and serve immediately

Asian Style Cauliflower Rice

I've been making tons of varieties of cauliflower rice, but this version with a bunch of veggies including edamame, spinach and bell peppers is one of my favorites. I love the vegetables in the recipe, but you can add baby boy choy, grated carrots, chopped broccoli or anything else you have on hand. Everything in the recipe should be chopped so it cooks really quick making it a quick meal to whip up. I totally suggest making double as it's great to eat right out of the fridge the next day for a �uick, low carb lunch.

Ingredients

- 2 tablespoons olive oil
- 1 onion, finely diced
- 1 yellow or orange bell pepper, seeded and diced
- 1 head cauliflower, chopped in food processor until it resembles rice
- 2 teaspoons fresh ginger, minced
- 3 cups fresh spinach, roughly chopped
- 1 cup shelled edamame

- 3 tablespoons low sodium soy sauce
- 1/2 teaspoon kosher salt
- 2 scallions, chopped

Preparation

1. Heat a large wok or sauté pan over medium heat, add oil and sauté onion and ginger for 1 minute. Add bell pepper and cook for 1 minute.

2. Add cauliflower and cook for an additional 2-3 minutes. Add spinach, edamame, soy sauce and salt. Cook for 3-4 minutes or until cauliflower is tender.

3. Top with chopped scallions and serve.

Smoked Salmon Scramble

This recipe comes together ⍰uickly so it makes a great protein-rich breakfast on busy school mornings. Or serve it with orange juice, bagels, and fresh fruit for a leisurely weekend brunch the whole family will enjoy.

Ingredients

• 8 large eggs

• 4 chives, chopped

• 1/2 teaspoon kosher salt

• 2 teaspoons canola oil or butter

• 4 pieces thinly sliced smoked salmon, chopped

Preparation

1. In a bow, whisk together the eggs, chives, and salt.

2. Heat the oil or butter in a sauté pan over medium heat.

3. Add the egg mixture to the pan, and cook, stirring occasionally until almost set, about 4 minutes.

4. Stir in the salmon and continue to cook for 1 minute longer.

Japanese Sticky Chicken

Japanese Sticky Chicken is packed with flavor and perfect for anyone wanting an easy to prepare, family friendly meal!

This Japanese Sticky Chicken has a sweet and salty taste that begs to be eaten with your hands and tastes finger lickin' good. I've made it 5 times with slight variations, so I've had plenty of leftovers that were just as tasty as when the chicken first came out of the oven. Serve it with Perfect Brown Rice and my kids new re?uest of a wedge of salad topped with Carrot Ginger Miso and you've got the perfect summer meal!

Ingredients

- 1 tablespoon minced fresh ginger
- 1/4 cup mirin
- 1/4 cup honey
- 1/4 cup low sodium soy sauce
- 1 tablespoon rice vinegar
- 1 tablespoon sesame oil

- 1 teaspoon togarashi spice blend, optional
- 2 bone-in, skin-on chicken breasts
- 4 bone-in, skin-on chicken legs
- 3 scallions, chopped

Preparation

1. In a large zipper bag or in 13 x 9 baking dish, whisk the first 7 ingredients.

2. Add the chicken to the sauce, turning the pieces so they are completely coated. Marinate 1 hour in the refrigerator or up to overnight.

3. Preheat the oven to 450F.

4. Bake Chicken, skin side up, for 30 minutes or until golden brown.

5. Serve sprinkled with scallions

Salmon BLT Salad with Chive Ranch Dressing

This Salmon BLT Salad is a family favorite and perfect for summer grilling or anytime of year! Perfectly seasoned salmon is either pan fried or grilled and layered with greens, crispy bacon, avocados and tossed in a Whole30 compliant chive ranch dressing. It's paleo, low carb, and keto friendly too!

Ingredients

Dressing:

- 1/4 cup plain unsweetened almond milk
- 1/2 cup paleo mayo homemade or store bought
- 1 Tbsps lemon juice
- 1 tsp fresh minced dill or 1/4 tsp dried
- 1 garlic clove minced
- 2 Tbsp chopped chives
- Sea Salt & black pepper to taste

Salmon:

- 1 lb individual salmon fillets skin on or off (3-4 fillets)

• 3/4 tsp garlic powder

• 3/4 tsp onion powder

• 3/4 tsp smoked paprika

• 3/4 tsp sea salt

• 1/8 teaspoon black pepper

• 1 Tbsp bacon fat avocado oil, or ghee

Salad:

• 6 cups mixed greens of choice roughly chopped

• 1 cup cherry tomatoes halved

• 6 Slices bacon cooked until crisp and crumbled or chopped

• 1 medium avocado thinly sliced

• 1 small red onion thinly sliced

Instructions

Dressing:

1. Whisk together the almond milk, mayo, lemon juice and dill until smooth. Stir in the garlic and chives, then season to taste with sea salt and black pepper.

Salmon:

1. Pat the fillets dry with paper towel. In a small bowl, mix together all the seasonings. You can make the salmon on the stovetop in a skillet or on the grill. If grilling, brush generously all over with the oil before beginning. If pan frying, the oil is for the skillet.

2. Heat the grill or skillet to medium high heat. Add oil to the skillet. In a skillet, place the salmon skin side down (if you chose skin) and cook about 3 minutes on each side, adjusting for preference and thickness.

3. If grilling, brush grill with oil and place the salmon flesh side down on the hot grill. Cook about 3 minutes, then carefully flip and cook skin side down for another 3-4 minutes, adjusting for thickness and preference.

4. Remove to a plate and assemble the salad. Layer the greens with tomatoes, bacon, sliced avocado and red onion and place salmon on top. Drizzle all over with as

much of the dressing as you like and garnish with extra chives if desired. Serve right away. Enjoy!

Garlic Butter Steak Bites

Tender steak seasoned with garlic, butter, and fresh herbs will be your new favorite weeknight dinner! This simple recipe only takes twenty minutes to make!

Ingredients

- ½ tablespoon avocado oil
- 2 pounds of steak, cut into small bite size pieces
- 2 teaspoons salt
- ½ teaspoon freshly ground black pepper
- ½ teaspoon red pepper flakes (optional)
- 2 tablespoons butter or ghee
- 6 cloves minced garlic
- ¼ cup chopped parsley
- green onion, for garnish

Method

1. Season the steak bites with salt, pepper, and red pepper flakes and stir until well coated.

2. Heat a large skillet over medium-high heat. Add the avocado oil to the hot skillet and then add the steak in a single layer. Cook the steak bites for 3-4 minutes until brown, stirring occasionally. You may have to do this in batches depending on the size of your skillet. Once the steak is brown, remove it from the pan.

3. Remove any excess water from the skillet and then add the butter or ghee to the pan. Next add the garlic and saute for 1 minute.

4. Add the steak back to the pan and cook for 1-2 minutes stirring to coat it in the butter sauce. Remove the pan from the heat and stir in the chopped parsley. Garnish with green onion and serve immediately.

Grilled Chicken Cobb Salad with Honey Dijon

This grilled chicken Cobb salad is packed with all the goodies! Perfectly seasoned grilled chicken, crispy bacon, sliced eggs and avocado plus an easy and delicious honey dijon dressing that's ready in under a minute! This Cobb salad makes a healthy, hearty, low carb meal that's gluten free, paleo, dairy free and a family favorite!

Ingredients

Dressing:

- 3 Tbsp raw honey melted (if solid)
- 1/4 cup dijon mustard
- 2 Tbsp fresh lemon juice or white vinegar
- 1/4 cup avocado oil
- 1/4 tsp sea salt

Salad:

- 3-4 boneless skinless chicken breasts about 1 1/2 lbs
- 1 tsp sea salt
- 1/2 tsp black pepper

- 1/2 tsp garlic powder
- 1/2 tsp onion powder
- 1 Tbsp avocado oil for the grill or pan
- 8 cups chopped romaine kale, or other greens, or a mix
- 3/4 cup cherry tomatoes halved
- 1/2 red onion thinly sliced
- 1 med cucumber peeled and sliced
- 1 large avocado thinly sliced
- 8 slices bacon cooked until crisp, and chopped or crumbled*
- 6 hard boiled eggs sliced**

Instructions

Dressing:

1. You can either whisk the dressing together in a bowl, streaming in the oil slowly until well combined, or use an immersion blender. If using the blender, place all ingredients in a tall jar and blend until well combined. I

like to use an immersion blender for a thicker, smoother dressing. Once done, set aside or refrigerate to use later.

Salad:

1. Combine the salt, pepper, garlic and onion powder in a small bowl and season the chicken all over. Heat your grill (or a grill pan) to medium/med-high heat and brush with the oil. Once sizzling hot, add chicken and grill about 5 minutes per side or until just cooked through. Internal temperature of the chicken should reach 165°F. Remove to a cutting board and set aside.

2. In a large serving bowl, layer the salad greens with the tomatoes, red onion, cucumber, avocado, cooked and crumbled bacon, and sliced hardboiled eggs. Thinly slice the grilled chicken and layer into the salad as desired. Drizzle the dressing over the top and toss, or serve it on the side. Enjoy!

Shrimp Fried Cauliflower Rice

This shrimp fried cauliflower rice tastes just like the real thing (maybe better!) but it's healthier and easy to make at home! Loaded with flavor, protein, veggies and healthy fats, it makes a great weeknight meal that everyone will love – even the picky kiddos! Paleo, Whole30 compliant, and keto friendly.

Ingredients

- 1 lb medium-large raw shrimp peeled and deveined
- 1 tsp tapioca flour or arrowroot*
- Sea salt and black pepper
- 2 Tbsp avocado oil or ghee divided
- 3 eggs whisked
- 1 1/2 cups carrots diced
- 1 bunch scallions white and green parts separated - thinly sliced
- 1-inch chunk fresh ginger peeled and minced about 2 tsp
- 3 cloves garlic minced

• 12 oz cauliflower rice fresh or frozen. If frozen, thaw first.

• 1/4 cup coconut aminos (this is a paleo and Whole30 friendly e⍰uivalent of soy sauce)

• 1 tbsp pure sesame oil

• Sea salt to taste

Instructions

1. Have all ingredients prepped and ready to go before beginning.

2. In a bowl, toss the shrimp with the tapioca or arrowroot, salt and pepper. Heat a large nonstick skillet over medium high heat. Once hot, add 1 Tbsp avocado oil or ghee. Add shrimp in a single layer and cook 1-2 minutes per side until opa⍰ue, careful not to overcook. Remove to a plate and turn the heat to medium.

3. With the skillet over medium heat, add the whisked eggs and cook until just set, breaking them up with your spatula. Set them aside with the shrimp.

4. Add the second tablespoon of oil or ghee to the skillet and adjust heat medium high. Add the diced carrots and cook, stirring, 3-4 minutes or until fork tender. Then add in the white part of the scallions, ginger, and garlic and stir to combine. Cook another minute until fragrant.

5. Add in the cauliflower rice, coconut aminos and sesame oil and stir to combine. Cook about 2-3 minutes to soften the cauliflower rice. Add in the shrimp and eggs and stir and cook 30-60 seconds to heat through, then remove from heat. Garnish with the green part of the scallions and additional coconut aminos or salt and pepper to taste. Serve right away. Leftovers can be saved in the sealed container in the refrigerator for up to 4 days. Enjoy!

Cajun Shrimp and Sausage Skillet

This cajun shrimp and sausage skillet is made with flavor andouille sausage, protein packed shrimp, and crisp bell peppers. This recipe is an easy weeknight meal that will take you only ten minutes from start to finish making. Serve it with your favorite sides for a delicious, healthy, and filling meal that everyone will love!

Ingredients

- 2 tablespoons avocado oil or ghee
- 12 oz andouille sausage, sliced
- 1 tablespoon finely minced garlic
- 1 small red bell pepper, sliced
- 1 small green bell pepper, sliced
- 1 small orange bell pepper, sliced
- 1/2 yellow onion, sliced
- 1/4 cup sliced green onion
- 1 pound shrimp, peeled and deveined
- 1/2 tablespoon cajun seasoning (plus more to taste)

- juice of one lemon
- salt and pepper to taste

Method

1. Heat a large skillet over medium-high heat. Once the skillet is hot, add in the avocado oil or ghee.

2. Add the minced garlic and cook for minute until fragrant.

3. Add the sliced andouille sausage and cook for three to four minutes to brown on both sides. When the sausage has browned, add the sliced bell peppers and onions to the skillet. Season with salt, pepper, and the cajun seasoning. Cook the veggies for three to four minutes.

4. Next, add the shrimp to the skillet and toss to combine. Cook for two to three minutes until the shrimp is translucent and cooked through.

5. Remove the skillet from the heat and add the lemon juice, sliced green onion, and more seasoning to taste. Serve immediately.

Spaghetti S⍰uash Bolognese

This easy spaghetti s⍰uash bolognese is great for healthy weeknight dinners with a flavorful meat sauce and perfectly roasted “al dente” spaghetti s⍰uash! It’s dairy-free, Whole30 compliant, paleo, gluten free and Low FODMAP too. Perfect to prep ahead of time and the leftovers are delicious!

Ingredients

• 1 medium spaghetti s⍰uash

• Avocado oil or avocado oil spray

• Sea salt and black pepper

• 1 large carrot peeled and finely diced

• 2 large stalk celery finely diced

• 2 Tbsp garlic infused oil Fody Foods, or other

• 4 slices bacon turkey bacon is fine too

• 1 lb grass fed ground beef OR 1/2 lb ground pork and 1/2 lb ground beef

• Sea salt and black pepper

• 1/4 tsp oregano

• 2 cups low FODMAP marinara sauce Fody Foods or Rao's sensitive

• 1/3 cup coconut milk full fat (optional)

• Fresh parsley or basil for garnish

Instructions

For the S⍰uash:

1. Preheat your oven to 400°F and line a baking sheet with parchment paper. Cut the squash in half lengthwise and scoop out the seeds and strings. Spray the inside of the squash with avocado oil spray or brush with oil, and sprinkle with sea salt and black pepper.

2. Place s⍰uash face down on the baking sheet and roast in the preheated oven for 20-25 minutes, depending on size and preference for softness. I prefer my squash al dente and roast for about 20-22 minutes. You can press down gently on the back of the s⍰uash to see if it’s tender.

For the Sauce:

1. While the squash roasts, heat a large skillet over medium-hi heat and add the garlic infused oil. Once heated, add the carrot and celery to the skillet and cook until tender - about 3 minutes. Add the bacon to the skillet and cook, stirring, until about 3/4 of the way done. If the bacon renders a lot of fat, you can drain some at this point (optional).

2. Crumble the ground meat into the skillet and sprinkle with sea salt, black pepper and the oregano. Cook, stirring, to brown.

3. Once the meat is browned and the bacon crisp, add in the tomato basil or marinara sauce and the coconut milk, if using. Bring to a boil while stirring occasionally, then lower the heat and simmer for 5-10 more minutes to thicken and allow the flavors to blend.

4. Use a fork to scrape the "spaghetti" strands from the squash and place in a serving bowl. Serve topped with the Bolognese sauce and garnish with parsley or basil if desired. Enjoy!

Broccoli Slaw & Spicy Shrimp Salad

This recipe is very personal and versatile. If you aren't a fan of shrimp or shellfish in general, you can always use the same rub we used for the shrimp to season up some chicken or pork and pair that with the slaw. You can also switch up the ingredients in the slaw. As you will see if the full recipe below, we added purple onions, sweet mini bell peppers, cilantro, cherry tomatoes, and bacon pieces. However, the ingredients list is completely customizable. You can switch things up and add your own favorite vegetables. Or you don't eat bacon, omit it and just finish the salad with the shrimp, chicken, fish or whatever you choose.

Ingredients

Scale

1 lb. wild-caught shrimp (peeled and deveined)

1 tsp. old bay seasoning

1/2 tsp. ground turmeric

1/4 tsp. cayenne pepper

1/2 tsp. garlic powder

1 tbsp. grass-fed ghee

1 tbsp. lemon juice

1/2 a purple onion (sliced)

1 12- ounce pack of broccoli slaw

5 sweet mini bell peppers (julienned)

2 tbsp. freshly chopped cilantro (or parsley)

1 cup cherry tomatoes

3 slices cooked no sugar added bacon

DRESSING:

1/2 a cup avocado mayo

2 tbsp. yellow mustard

1 1/2 tsp. lemon juice

1/4 tsp. garlic powder

1/4 tsp. cracked black pepper

1 tbsp. filtered water

Instructions

To begin, pat the shrimp dry and toss them with the old bay seasoning, turmeric, cayenne pepper, and garlic powder. Now, heat the ghee over medium-high heat in a large skillet. Add the shrimp to the pan and sear for ~3 minutes on both sides or until the shrimp is pink. Remove the shrimp from the heat, toss with 1 tablespoon of lemon juice and set them aside.

Now, add the broccoli slaw, purple onions, bell peppers, cilantro, tomatoes and bacon to a large mixing bowl and aside.

Now, add all of the ingredients needed for the dressing to a small mixing bowl and whisk until creamy.

Add the dressing to the broccoli slaw mixture and toss to combine. Season with a couple pinches of sea salt to your desired taste. Transfer the salad to a serving dish and finish with the spicy shrimp. Garnish with lemon wedges and enjoy!

Paleo Egg Roll in a Bowl with Chicken

Simple yet incredibly delicious, these Paleo Egg Roll Bowls with Chicken are bound to become a new go-to for you! An easy stir fry that tastes just like an egg roll topped with a sesame aioli that you'll want to put on everything!

Ingredients

Sesame Aioli:

- 1/2 cup homemade mayo or purchased paleo mayo
- 2 cloves garlic minced, or 1 tsp garlic powder
- 2 tsp sesame oil
- 1 1/2 tsp lime juice
- 3 tsp hot sauce Whole30 compliant

Egg Roll Bowls:

- 1 1/2 lbs boneless skinless chicken thighs cut into pieces or strips
- 1 1/2 Tbsp avocado oil divided
- Sea salt and pepper for the chicken

- 1/2 tsp onion powder
- Pinch cayenne pepper optional
- 6-7 cups shredded veggies slaw mixture or a combination of shredded cabbage, carrots, brussels sprouts
- 3 tbsp coconut aminos
- 1 1/2 Tbsp sesame oil
- 1 tsp hot sauce Whole30 compliant, optional
- 1 bunch scallions thinly sliced white/light green and green parts separated
- 3 cloves garlic minced
- 2 tsp ginger fresh, about 1” peeled and grated or minced

Instructions

Prepare Aioli

1. Whisk together the mayo, garlic, sesame oil, lime or lemon juice, hot sauce, and cayenne, if using until smooth, refrigerate until ready to use.

Stir fry the Chicken and veggies:

1. Have all ingredients prepped and ready to go before beginning since the cooking will go fast.

2. Heat a large nonstick skillet or wok over high heat and add 1 Tbsp of the oil. Sprinkle the chicken with salt, pepper, onion powder, and a dash of cayenne pepper if desired.

3. Once skillet is smoking hot, add the chicken and cook, stirring to brown evenly, for about 5 minutes or until browned and cooked through, then remove to a plate while you cook veggies.

4. Lower heat to med and add 1/2 Tbsp of oil. Add the slaw/shredded veggies, cook and stir for about a minute until beginning to soften, then add the white scallions, ginger and garlic.

5. Cook another minute, then add the coconut aminos, sesame oil, and hot sauce, if using, to the skillet and stir, add the chicken back in, stir to combine well. Remove from heat and garnish with sliced green onion.

6. Serve in bowls drizzled with the spicy aioli*. Enjoy!

Low-Carb Chinese Beef and Noodles

Forget takeout. This �uick and easy Asian noodles will hit the spot every time. Zucchini noodles with a rich sweet and spicy beef sauce.

Ingredients

4 medium zucchinis

1 tbsp. Avocado oil

1 tbsp. Pure Sesame seed oil

2 garlic cloves – finely minced

1 onion – sliced

salt and pepper

1 lb. pasture raised ground beef

SAUCE:

4 tbsp. Coconut aminos

2 tbsp. Unsweetened applesauce

1 tsp. Korean pepper flakes (or crushed red pepper flakes)

1 tbsp. Unsweetened BBQ sauce

TO SERVE:

The greens of 2 scallions – chopped

sesame seeds (about a tablespoon)

Instructions

First, spiralize all 4 zucchinis and transfer the noodles to a large bowl lined with a clean kitchen towel and a large sheet of cheesecloth. Sprinkle on a few pinches of salt and set the noodles aside.

Then, add all the ingredients needed for the sauce into a small bowl and whisk to combine. Set the sauce aside.

Heat a large deep skillet over medium-high heat and add the avocado and sesame oils. Add the onions and garlic to the pan and sauté until the onions are tender and the garlic is fragrant, about 3-5 minutes while stirring continuously. Season the onion and garlic with a little salt and pepper. Push the onion and garlic to one side of the pan and add the ground beef to the skillet. Use a potato masher to break up the beef. Continue to cook the ground beef until it's browned, about 3-5 minutes.

Slowly add the sauce to the ground beef mixture and stir to combine. Turn the heat up a bit and continue to cook the mixture until the meat begins to caramelize a bit.

Now, s⍰ueeze as much li⍰uid out the zucchini noodles as you possibly can and add the noodles to the skillet with the beef mixture. Stir the noodles in with the beef mixture until all the flavors marry and the noodles are warm through, about 2-3 minutes. At this point, you can taste and add more salt if needed (but you shouldn't need any more salt).

Finish the beef and noodles with fresh scallions and sesame seeds. Serve immediately.

Sausage and Bell Pepper Skillet

This Sausage and Bell Pepper Skillet pretty much the easiest of easiest 5-Ingredient weeknight meals. Aside from the minimal ingredient list, the actual process of putting this together and getting it on the table is pretty much the easiest thing ever.

Ingredients

- 2 tbsp extra virgin olive oil
- 1 lb Italian Sausage, cut into 2 inch pieces
- 2 bell peppers, seeded and sliced thin (I use one red and one green. But any are fine)
- 1/2 yellow onion, sliced thin
- kosher salt, to taste
- black pepper, to taste
- 1 cup store bought marinara
- 2 cups baby arugula, for serving

Instructions

1. Heat oil in a large skillet over medium-high heat.

2. Add the cut sausages to the skillet and brown on both sides, 2-3 minutes per side. Transfer brown sausages to a plate and set aside.

3. Add the sliced bell peppers and onions to the skillet with some salt and pepper and cook, stirring, until tender, 4 to 6 minutes.

4. Pour in the marinara and stir to combine. Nestle the sausages into the sauce and let simmer to reheat the sausages, about 3 more minutes.

5. Serve over a bed of arugula, enjoy!

Korean-inspired Ground Beef and Kimchi Bowls

These Korean-inspired Ground Beef and Kimchi Bowls are far from authentic, but it's a fun Korean-inspired easy weeknight dish that packs on zing with very little effort. All you really have to do is brown some meat with a few added aromatics, serve with some prepared cauliflower rice, store-bought kimchi, and a little fresh crunch of cucumber and BAM! Dinner is served. Easy!!

Ingredients

For the Ground Beef:

- 2 tbsp coconut aminos
- 1 tsp toasted sesame oil
- 1/2 tsp finely grated ginger
- 1 tbsp peeled and finely grated pear
- 1 tsp fish sauce
- 2 tbsp rice vinegar
- 2 cloves of garlic, minced
- 1/4 tsp crushed red pepper flakes (optional)

- 1 tbsp olive oil
- 1 lb ground beef
- 1/2 tsp kosher salt
- 1/2 tsp black pepper

For the Cauliflower Rice

- 3 cups riced cauliflower
- 1 tsp olive oil

For Serving:

- 1 cup store-bought kimchi I like Wildbrine
- 1/2 english cucumber, thinly sliced
- 2 tbsp fresh cilantro leaves
- toasted sesame seeds optional
- black sesame seeds optional

Instructions

For the Ground Beef:

1. Combine coconut aminos, toasted sesame oil, ginger, pear, fish sauce, rice vinegar, garlic and crushed red pepper flakes. Whisk until well combined. Set aside.

2. In a large skillet over medium high heat, heat olive oil. Add the ground beef, salt and pepper and break up with the back of spoon. Cook until the beef is cooked through, no longer pink, about 5-7 minutes.

3. Drain off the excess fat then add the beef back to skillet with the prepared sauce. Cook, stirring, until the sauce reduces and coats the meat, about 4 minutes.

4. Remove from heat. Cover to keep warm and set aside.

For the Cauliflower Rice:

1. In a separate skillet over medium heat, add the olive oil and cauliflower rice until the cauliflower is heated through. About 3 minutes.

For the Bowls:

1. To serve, Divide desired amount of beef in two bowls alongside the prepared cauliflower rice. Serve along side

kimchi and top with sliced cucumber and fresh cilantro. Garnish with sesame seeds, if desired. Enjoy!

Instant Pot Buffalo Chicken Casserole

This Instant Pot Buffalo Chicken Casserole is a simple 5-ingredient Whole30 and Keto meal! Tender chicken, buffalo sauce cauliflower rice, broccoli, and dairy free cream cheese make for the best combo! It comes together in 20 minutes and can also be made in the slow cooker.

Ingredients

- ▢ 1.5 lbs boneless skinless chicken breasts, I used 3 chicken breasts
- ▢ 1 bottle sugar free buffalo sauce, Primal Kitchen, Tessemae's, or The New Primal will all work!
- ▢ 1 12 oz bag broccoli florets
- ▢ 1 tbsp olive oil
- ▢ 1 16 oz package frozen cauliflower rice
- ▢ 1 tub Kite Hill chive almond milk cream cheese, can sub regular cream cheese if you tolerate dairy

Instructions

• Preheat your oven to 415. Add the broccoli florets to a parchment lined baking sheet and toss with olive oil. Add salt and pepper to taste. Bake for 12 minutes.

• Add the chicken breasts to your instant pot and pour the entire bottle of buffalo sauce on top. Toss the breasts so they are coated and some of the sauce is touching the bottom of the pot. This will prevent the burn notice from happening! Cook the chicken on manual high pressure for 12 minutes.

• While the chicken is cooking, cook the cauliflower rice. This can be done in the microwave if you have a microwavable frozen bag, or on the stove.

• When the chicken is done cooking, manually release the steam. Shred the chicken using two forks. Add in the cooked cauliflower rice and tub of Kite Hill cream cheese. Stir to combine. Add in the cooked broccoli and stir. Serve topped with Tessemae's ranch dressing, if desired. Enjoy!

Slow Cooker Instructions

• Add the chicken and buffalo sauce to your slow cooker. Cook on high for 3-4 hours or low for 7-8 hours. During the last 15 minutes of cooking time, cook the broccoli and cauliflower rice according to the directions above. Shred the chicken using two forks, then combine everything. Stir well and serve with ranch dressing, if desired. Enjoy!

Creamy Tuscan Chicken

This creamy paleo tuscan chicken is a super-tasty one-skillet meal that's perfect for weeknights and full of flavor! Boneless, skinless chicken thighs are seared and cooked with a creamy sauce packed with spinach and sun-dried tomatoes. Paleo, dairy-free, Whole30, and Keto friendly!

Ingredients

- 1.5 lbs chicken thighs boneless and skinless
- 1 Tbsp coconut oil plus additional if needed
- Sea salt and pepper
- 1/4 tsp garlic powder
- 1/4 tsp onion powder
- 1 small onion chopped
- 4 cloves garlic minced
- 1 Tbsp tapioca flour or arrowroot
- 1 cup chicken bone broth
- 1/2 cup coconut milk full fat, blended before adding if needed

• 1/2 Tbsp stone ground mustard

• 1 1/2 Tbsp nutritional yeast optional

• 1 tsp Italian seasoning blend

• 1/4 tsp sea salt or to taste

• 1/8 tsp black pepper or to taste

• 2/3 cup sun dried tomatoes roughly chopped

• 1 1/2 cups baby spinach roughly chopped

Instructions

1. Season the chicken with sea salt, pepper, garlic, and onion powder. In a large skillet add the coconut oil and cook the chicken thighs on medium-high heat for 5-7 minutes on each side or until browned and no longer pink in center. Remove chicken and set aside on a plate.

2. Add additional oil if necessary and cook the onions over medium heat until soft, then stir in the garlic and cook another 45 seconds.

3. Whisk in the tapioca or arrowroot, the add the broth and coconut milk. Stir to combine, then stir in the mustard, yeast, Italian seasoning, sea salt and pepper.

Cook and stir over medium-high heat until it starts to thicken.

4. Add the spinach and sun-dried tomatoes and allow mixture to simmer until spinach is wilted and tomatoes are softened. Add chicken back to the skillet and simmer another 2 minutes. Serve over cauli rice, zucchini noodles, or with roasted potatoes. Enjoy!

Grilled Balsamic Chicken with Peaches

am absolutely in love with this meal! Grilled Balsamic Chicken with Peaches was something that I did not know I needed in my life, but now that it's here, it is here to stay! The chicken is so flavorful and juicy, and the peaches are so tender and sweet. It is a match made in heaven!

Ingredients

• 1/2 cup of balsamic vinegar

• 2 tbsp of coconut aminos

• 2 tbsp of olive oil, plus more for coating the peaches and grill pan

• 1 tsp of granulated garlic

• 1 tsp of granulated onion

• 2 lbs of boneless and skinless chicken thighs

• 4 peaches, halved and seeded

• 4 green onions, sliced

• salt and pepper

Instructions

1. First make the marinade. Add balsamic vinegar, coconut aminos, olive oil, granulated garlic, granulated onion, and salt and pepper to a small mixing bowl. Whisk all of the ingredients together.

2. Add chicken thighs to a medium bowl and pour marinade over chicken. Ensure chicken is evenly coated in marinade. Refrigerate for at least 2 hours, but overnight is even better.

3. Remove chicken from the refrigerator when ready to start grilling peaches.

4. Heat a grill pan over medium-high heat. Bush both sides of peaches with olive oil and place cut-side down hot grill pan, about 4 minutes. Flip peaches and grill on skin-side until very soft, about another 4 minutes. Remove peaches from grill, add to a platter and set aside.

5. Carefully wipe down grill pan to remove any remnants from the peaches so it doesn't start to burn.

6. Next, add chicken thighs to hot grill and grill for about 8 minutes. Flip and cook for about 6 minutes, or until internal temperature reaches 165 degrees F. Remove chicken and add to platter with peaches.

7. Garnish with sliced green onions and serve.

Tandoori Chicken Burgers

These Indian inspired Tandoori Chicken Burgers are a flavourful way to switch up your usual burger. The tandoori flavoured chicken burgers are served with slices of cucumber, tomatoes, red onion and a delicious ginger and parsley sauce.

Ingredients

Tandoori Chicken Patties

o 1 pound ground chicken or turkey

o 3 cloves garlic minced

o 1/4 cup chopped cilantro

o 1 1/2 tbsp grated red onion

o 1 tbsp grated ginger

o 1 1/2 tbsp lemon juice

o 1/2 tsp lemon zest

o 1/2 tsp cayenne pepper

o 1 tsp cumin

o 1 tsp coriander

o 1 tsp paprika

o 1 tsp turmeric

o 1/2 tsp salt

o 1/2 tsp pepper

Ginger & Parsley Sauce

o 1/4 cup mayonnaise

o 1 tsp lemon juice

o 1/2 tbsp chopped mint

o 1 tbsp chopped parsley

o 1 tsp finely chopped ginger

o 1/4 tsp cumin

For Serving

o 1 head iceberg lettuce

o 1 large tomato thinly sliced

o 1/2 red onion thinly sliced

o 1/2 cucumber cut into thin slices or ribbons

Instructions

• In a bowl combine all of the ingredients for the tandoori chicken patties and use your hands to mix everything together so the spies are well incorporated in the meat. Divide the meat into 4 portions and form into patties.

• Heat a barbecue or grill pan on medium high heat. Grill the patties for 5 minutes per side until cooked through.

• While the patties are cooking, in a bowl combine all of the ingredients for the sauce and stir until well mixed. Set aside.

• Cut the iceberg lettuce into �uarters and separate each �uarter into two halves.

• To assemble the burgers spread the sauce on the inside of the lettuce. Top with 2 slices of red onion, sliced tomato and cucumber and place a tandoori patty on top. Place the other half of the lettuce leaf on top like a sandwich and wrap the burger in parchment paper to make it easier to eat.

Air Fryer Salmon Teriyaki

Air fryer salmon teriyaki recipe ready in 8 mins! The air fried salmon with teriyaki glaze is the best keto Teriyaki salmon when you want dinner fast!

Ingredients

- ▢ 1/3+1/4 cup Keto Teriyaki Sauce, see notes
- ▢ 16.5 oz. salmon fillets (3 slices at 5.5 oz per fillet), 1.5-inch at thickest
- ▢ 1/8 tsp xanthan gum
- ▢ Toasted white sesame seeds, sprinkle optional
- ▢ 1 bulb scallion, chopped

Instructions

For the teriyaki sauce:

- Follow these keto teriyaki sauce recipe instructions to prepare the sauce but do not add the xanthan gum thickener. Let the sauce cool to room temperature.

Loaded Bacon Burger Bowls

These deconstructed loaded bacon burger bowls have all the goodies you love in a burger! Sautéed mushrooms and onions, crispy bacon, pickles, tomatoes, red onion and a "cheesy" ranch sauce! Paleo, Whole30, and keto friendly and seriously delicious!

Ingredients

"Cheesy" Ranch Sauce:

- 2/3 cup homemade mayo or purchased paleo mayo
- 1 Tbsp coconut milk or almond milk
- 2 tsp lemon juice
- 2 tsp nutritional yeast for cheesy flavor
- 1/2 tsp garlic powder
- 1/2 tsp onion powder
- 2 tsp dried chives
- 1/8-1/4 tsp sea salt or to taste

Remaining Ingredients:

- 8 slices nitrate free bacon

- 1-2 Tbsp bacon fat or other cooking fat
- 1 medium onion diced
- 1 cup white mushrooms sliced
- 1 lb grass fed ground beef 85% lean
- Sea salt
- 1/4 tsp chipotle powder
- 1/4 tsp garlic powder
- Butter lettuce or greens of choice
- 1 cup cherry tomatoes
- Sliced dill pickles no added sugar
- Thinly sliced red onion
- Ranch sauce see above

Instructions

Ranch Sauce:

1. Whisk together all the ingredients in a small bowl and set aside or refrigerate until ready to use.

Burger Bowls:

1. In a large skillet, cook the bacon until crisp, remove to drain and cool. Reserve 1-2 Tbsp of the bacon fat and lower the heat to medium.

2. Add the onions to the hot skillet and cook until translucent, then add mushrooms and continue to cook until softened. Push veggies to the side and add the beef and sprinkle everything with sea salt, chipotle powder and garlic powder.

3. Stir beef to brown and mix in the with mushrooms and onions. Once beef is browned, remove from heat.

4. To assemble the bowls, layer your greens with the beef mixture, tomatoes, pickles, red onions, and bacon. Top with the ranch sauce and serve right away. Enjoy!

Beef and Broccoli Stir Fry

Healthy Beef and Broccoli Stir Fry is an easy ten minute meal that the whole family will love. Made with fresh and flavorful ingredients this copycat takeout recipe is so simple that you will never want to order takeout again. All you need are a few ingredients to make this healthier version of your favorite dish. Serve it over white rice or cauliflower for a full meal!

Ingredients

- 1 tablespoon avocado oil
- 1 pound steak, thinly sliced
- 4 cloves garlic, minced
- 1 teaspoon minced fresh ginger
- 1 teaspoon salt
- 1/4 teaspoon black pepper
- 1 teaspoon red pepper flakes
- 4 cups broccoli florets
- 1/3 cup water

• 1/4 cup coconut aminos

• 1 ½ teaspoon sesame oil

• 1/2 tablespoon arrowroot starch

• 1/4 cup green onion

• Sesame seeds, for garnish

Method

1. Add the sliced steak, garlic, ginger, salt, and pepper, to a mixing bowl and stir until well combined.

2. Heat a large skillet over medium-high heat. Once hot, add a tablespoon of avocado oil and then add in the steak. Cook the steak for 4-5 minutes until browned flipping halfway through. Once cooked, remove the steak from pan and set aside.

3. While the steak is cooking, make the stir fry sauce. Add the coconut aminos, sesame oil, red pepper, and arrowroot starch to a small bowl and whisk until well combined.

4. Once the steak has been removed from the pan, add in the broccoli florets and ⅓ cup of water. Cook the broccoli

until it is bright green and slightly tender but still has crunch; around 4-5 minutes depending on the size of the broccoli florets.

5. Add the steak and any juices back to the skillet and then add the stir fry sauce. Give everything a stir to combine steak, broccoli, and sauce and cook for one more minute. The sauce should thicken a bit as it heats.

6. Remove the skillet from the heat and stir in the sliced green onions. Garnish with sesame seeds and then serve the stir-fry immediately. Eat and enjoy!

Mandarin Orange Chicken Salad

Mandarin Orange Chicken Salad recipe is Paleo/Whole30. With sweet mandarins and crisp veggies, drizzled in a unbelievably delicious Asian peanut sauce.

Ingredients

- ▢ 4 cups shredded green cabbage
- ▢ 2 cups thinly sliced radicchio or purple cabbage
- ▢ 2 cups tatsoi, see notes
- ▢ 2 cups julienned carrots
- ▢ 0.5 lb cooked chicken breasts or thighs, diced
- ▢ 2 bulbs scallions, chopped
- ▢ 0.5 cup slivered almonds
- ▢ Coarse seas salt to taste
- ▢ 10.5 oz canned mandarin oranges, I use WholeFoods in pear juice
- ▢ Toasted white or black sesame seeds, optional

For the Asian peanut sauce/salad dressing: (makes 1 cup)

- ▢ ⅓ cup canned Mandarin orange juice
- ▢ 2 tbsp coconut aminos
- ▢ 3 tbsp almond butter, or cashew nut or sunflower seed butter
- ▢ 0.25 oz grated garlic
- ▢ 0.25 oz grated ginger
- ▢ 1.5 tbsp rice vinegar
- ▢ ⅓ cup olive oil

Instructions

- In a large salad mixing bowl, add ingredients from cabbage to almonds.
- Drizzle the salad dressing over the salad bowl. Toss and incorporate well. Season with salt to taste. Place the mandarin oranges on top. Sprinkle toasted sesame seeds, if using. Serve at room temperature or slightly chilled.

Paleo Burrito Bowls with Cauliflower Rice

These easy, filling, totally satisfying Paleo Burrito Bowls are packed with spicy seasoned ground beef, sautéed peppers and onions, cauliflower rice and a quick guacamole. Served over fried cauliflower rice with a kick for maximum flavor!

Ingredients

For the Rice:

- 12 oz cauli rice I purchased this pre-"riced"
- 1 Tbsp coconut oil or other cooking fat
- 1/2 tsp sea salt
- 1 Tbsp fresh lime juice
- 1 Tbsp jalapeño pepper minced
- 1/2 tsp onion powder
- 1/2 tsp garlic powder
- Dash chipotle powder

For the Beef:

- 1 lb grass fed ground beef 80-85% lean

- 1 Tbsp coconut oil or other cooking fat
- 1/2 tsp sea salt
- 3/4 tsp onion powder
- 3/4 tsp garlic powder
- 1 tsp cumin
- 3/4 tsp chili powder
- Chipotle powder To taste - I added a generous dash
- 2 Tbsp tomato paste
- 4 Tbsp water

Peppers & Onions:

- 1 large onion sliced thin
- 1 large red bell pepper sliced thin
- 1 Tbsp coconut oil or other cooking fat
- sprinkle of sea salt

Guacamole:

- 1 large ripe avocado or 2 small

• 2-3 Tbsp onion minced

• 1 clove garlic minced

• 1-2 Tbsp jalapeno peppers minced

• 1 1/2 Tbsp fresh lime juice

• 2 Tbsp chopped fresh cilantro plus more for garnish

Instructions

For Cauli Rice:

1. Heat a large skillet over medium heat and add coconut oil or other fat. Add the riced cauliflower and stir to coat. Cover skillet and cook for about 2-3 minutes to steam.

2. Uncover and stir, then add the jalapeño pepper, salt, seasonings and lime juice. Cook and stir another minute or two uncovered until you have desired texture, then remove from heat.

For Beef, Peppers, Onions:

1. Meanwhile in a separate skillet (or the same one after cooking the cauli rice) heat 1 tbsp coconut oil over medium high heat.

2. Crumble the beef into the skillet and break up lumps with a wooden spoon or spatula. Add the salt and all seasonings and cook, stirring occasionally until browned. Do not drain the fat. Lower heat to medium-low and add the tomato paste and water, stir to combine. Continue to cook and stir until thickened, then remove to a separate bowl.

3. Heat the same skillet over medium (keeping juices in skillet) and add 1 tbsp coconut oil. Add peppers and onions and stir to coat with fat. Sprinkle with a bit of sea salt to taste, and continue to cook, stirring occasionally, about 5 minutes or until softened and browning, then remove from heat.

4. To make the guacomole, mash together the avocado with the rest of the ingredients, adjusting seasonings to taste.

5. *To assemble the bowls, begin with the cauliflower rice, then layer the beef, peppers and onions, and guacamole. Garnish with more cilantro and a s�ueeze of lime juice if desired.Enjoy!

CONCLUSION

You could lose weight following a Paleolithic diet – and quickly, depending on how strictly you adhere to eating the foods from the allowed list and how much physical exercise you add to your daily routine.

In the long term, you have to be sure you're getting calcium and other nutrients you're missing by not having dairy products and certain grains. Some paleo-approved foods, such as salmon and spinach, contain calcium, so you have to be sure you're including them in your diet. It would be a good idea to check with a registered dietitian, too, to make sure you're meeting your calcium and other nutrient needs. On the whole, the paleo diet is not a bad choice, Holley says. If someone follows the diet by cutting out processed food, processed meats, and sugar-sweetened beverages and swaps them for more fruits, vegetables, and healthy fats, they're likely to see some health benefits.

www.ingramcontent.com/pod-product-compliance
Lightning Source LLC
LaVergne TN
LVHW052046160826
845678LV00015B/3122

* 9 7 9 8 3 6 1 6 1 2 3 1 4 *